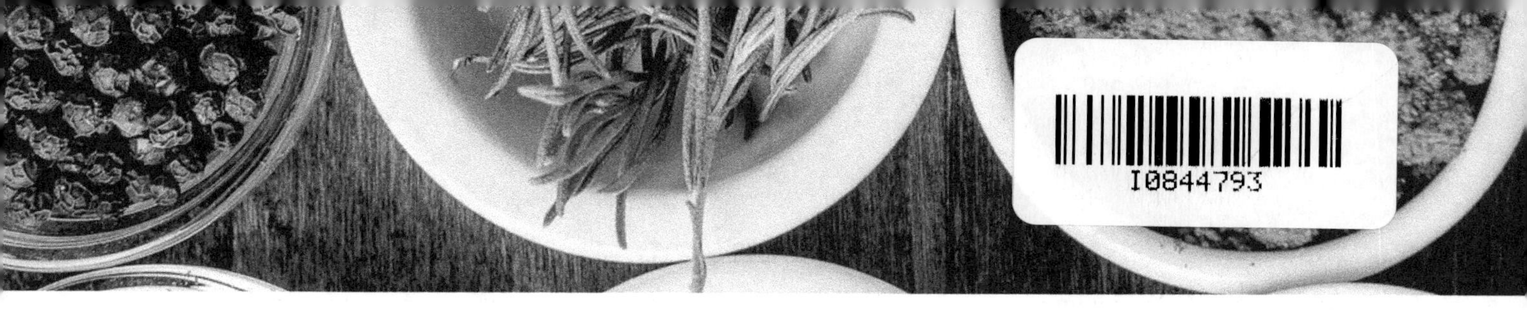

MEDICINAL

HERB

HANDBOOK

a beginner's guide

by Kerry Prince

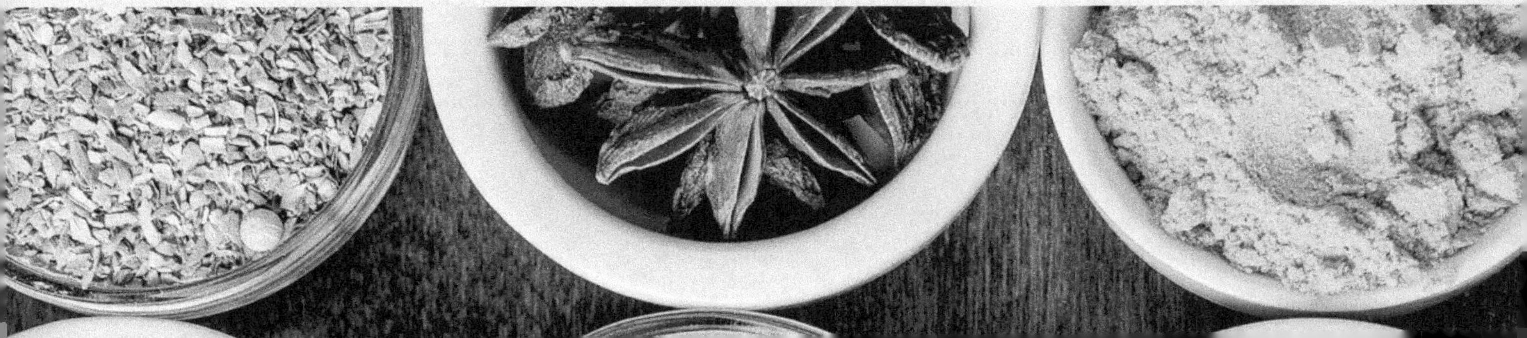

Contents

Introduction

Herbal medicine is a hot button topic and no longer considered a niche in the alternative health field. However, it isn't anything new, in fact it's as old as we are. A return to traditional plant therapy is becoming more mainstream as we recognize the multitude of side effects associated with pharmaceutical remedies.

The information in this e-book is a collection of many, many, many sources of information, consultations, classes and long talks with old healers. I don't claim to be an expert at all. I simply wish to share information that has helped me and many others. I encourage everyone reading this to let this be a spark to search for more information. There is a lot of information here, but it is only a fraction of the whole plant, so to speak.

Let me go ahead and get this out of the way. In no way is this book intended to replace a doctor's visit. Go to the doctor. There is sometimes a riff between those that believe in herbal remedies and those that follow what is referred to as "Western Medicine." There shouldn't be. Many medicines are derived from herbs and plants, so they can accompany many treatment plans. Conversely, they can also interfere. So, **please consult your physician before starting on any self-diagnosed treatment plan. Specifically, if you are pregnant, nursing or trying to get pregnant**.

HEALING THE WHOLE BODY vs. SYMPTOMS

Masking symptoms is an easy way to chase your health instead of being proactive. Herbs, like drugs, can be used to mask symptoms in the body. A better approach, in my opinion, is to see the whole person and treat the whole person. As opposed to seeing and treating specific conditions and diseases. Most herbal tonics are meant to strengthen the overall system, support health and vitality. Taken into account with exercise, lifestyle choices and a positive attitude; one can support a holistic approach to health by implementing plant-based remedies and tonics.

The body strives to be in balance. When you mask a symptom, you prevent the body from seeking equilibrium on its own. When done repeatedly you can drive the disorder deeper in the body. Which will eventually surface with a vengeance. Herbal therapies can help aid the body by supporting vitality and smoothly adapting the individual to daily stresses. Herbs have been touted for centuries to restore a person's sense of wellbeing, feeling nourished and balanced.

Often "symptoms" are the physical embodiment of the bodies healing process. For example. A cough. Coughing is a natural reflex of the body to expel excess mucus, allergens and bacteria from the respiratory tract. When you take something over the counter to quell the cough, yes you stop bothering people at work and your spouse can sleep. But you aren't doing much for yourself though. By taking expectorant herbs you'll facilitate movement and have more productive coughs.

Another great example is a fever. Impulsively we always try to bring the temperature down, right? A fever is the body's way of burning out the toxins making you sick. You can support this action by taking herbal remedies that support this action by allowing the blood to stay hot while cooling down the body. This is accomplished by opening the pores of the skin, promoting the release of heat and toxins through sweat.

One word you will see a lot in this book is "adaptogen." Its full definition is: *a natural substance considered to help the body adapt to stress and to exert a normalizing effect upon bodily processes.* In short, they help the body achieve the balance it desires. Becoming proactive with your health is key. Don't just refer to this book and other sources when something is wrong or doesn't feel right. Adaptogens and other nutritive herbs can help you perform "routine maintenance" that can help stave off illness and disease when accompanied with a healthy lifestyle.

A quick word on navigating the book. I have provided a list of **Single Plant Herbs** and what they have either been tested for, famous for or I personally vouch for. I have <u>underlined</u> some of my favorite herbs and ones I use daily. The **Herbal Combination** section is a collection of recipes tried and tested over many years. I have studied hundreds of combinations and found the ones most popular, most beneficial when combined and least likely to interfere with each other. The **Organ System Disorder** chapter isn't meant to replace your doctor (I can't say this enough) but to give you guidance and a quick reference.

CAUTIONS AND CONSIDERATIONS

1. I've said it already and I'll say it again. CONSULT YOUR PHYSICIAN. Especially if you are pregnant, nursing or planning a pregnancy.
2. Be careful of interactions with medications. Again. Consult a physician if you are currently on a treatment plan.
3. Only buy herbs in bulk from a trusted source and if you have a plan to store, freeze or make bulk oils/tinctures. Herbs can lose potency if stored incorrectly.
4. For herbs to act quickly, they need to be taken on an empty stomach.
5. "If a little is good, more is better"; doesn't typically translate to herbs. Especially for concentrated formulas.
6. Use common sense and listen to your body. If conditions get worse when you administer an herb, or you feel an allergic reaction. Stop. Then go see a doctor.

As I stated earlier, this isn't close to all there is to know about herbal medicine. I just hope this encourages you to continue learning and searching for balance and good health.

To Good Health,

Kerry Prince
Kerry In The Kitchen

SINGLE PLANTS

Agrimony-Useful in urinary tract infections and overactive or hypermetabolic liver from chemotherapy or drug excess.

Aletris-Has been shown to aid digestion and low back pain associated with pelvic prolapse or congestion.

Alfalfa-Nutritive herb that has a high mineral content that is easily digestible, particularly calcium, vitamin K, and folic acid, stimulates lactation while increasing the quality of breast milk

Angelica-Used in weak digestion; as an anti-spasmodic, it prevents uterine and intestinal cramping and regulates menses due to hormonal balancing properties.

Arnica- (External use only) Joint inflammation, sprains and sore muscles. Decreases swelling and bruising. Shown to help with arthritis.

Arrowroot-Digestive aid, treats urinary tract infection, boosts immune function and soothes gum and mouth pain. Common ingredient in teething cookies for babies.

Asafoetida-Asthma relief, lowers blood pressure, helps with IBS, gas reliever.

Ashwagandha-Improves thyroid function, reduces adrenal fatigue, combats stress and balances blood sugar levels. All around powerhouse herb.

Aspen-Anti-inflammatory and fever reducer. Aspirin like effects without the stomach irritation.

Astragalus-High level adaptogen. Strong anti-inflammatory, immune booster, antioxidant.

Bacopa-Adaptogen. Aids in cognition, memory and anxiety.

Baptisia-Blood cleansing properties for septic conditions. Stimulates metabolism of waste products and cellular repair. USE WITH CARE

Barberry-Good for liver, gallstones, ulcers and jaundice. Lowers fevers and blood pressure, acts as intestinal strengthener and laxative.

Bayberry-Topically, as gargle or douche, it reduces swollen tissue in gingivitis, tonsillitis, vaginitis and discharges.

Benzoin-Expectorant. Makes a nice steam in vaporizer or bath.

Betony-Relaxes muscles, decreases muscular pain and muscle spasms. Also used as a mild sedative.

Black Cohosh-Effective for cramping, hot flashes, aids in sleep. Studies have shown effectiveness treating uterine fibroids and PCOS.

Black Walnut-Works well for diarrhea and constipation. Anti-fungal. Aids with oil-soluble vitamin and B12 absorption.

Blessed Thistle-Stimulates digestive activity and is used to treat gastritis and peptic ulcers. Also used for estrogen deficiency and to stimulate lactation.

Blue Cohosh-Helpful in uterine infections by increasing fluid drainage. It will initiate a late period and decrease cramping.

Blue Flag-"Liver lymphatic", meaning it specifically deals with the draining of lymph from the liver. Gets natural oils to the skin and is good mixed with other herbs for toxicity. Increases perspiration and powerful liver stimulant.

Blue Vervain-Acid indigestion and heartburn. Has been used for children and adults with the flu.

Boneset-Aids with flu symptoms, expectorant.

Boswelia-Lowers inflammation, reduces joint and arthritis pain, speeds healing from infection.

Brickella-Decreases liver overproduction of glucose. Specific for adults with diabetes.

Bupleurum-Liver detoxifier, boosts adrenal gland function.

Burdock-Alkalinizes and eliminates toxins in the bloodstream. Used to treat chronic acne and psoriasis. Strengthens lymphatic system.

Calendula-Antioxidant and anti-inflammatory. Calms muscle spasms, increases blood flow and oxygen to wounds, improves oral health.

Cascara Sagrada-Used for chronic constipation, indigestion and hemorrhoids, helpful in gallstones and liver ailments.

Cat's Claw-Immune system enhancer. Used for arthritis, allergies and systemic candida. Increases circulation, lowers blood pressure and helps the body fight infection.

Cayenne-Best taken at the beginning of a cold. Helpful in stomach and lower bowel pain. Improves circulation. Use sparingly of course.

Chamomile-Acid indigestion and gas. Has been shown to help with morning sickness and general nausea.

Chaparral-Tones the liver and increases dietary fat metabolism. Pulls heavy metals from the body.

Chaparro Amargosa- For gastroenteritis, giardia, parasites, fungal infections, chronic digestive inflammation, stomach ulcers, post-antibiotic therapy, candida imbalance, drinking suspect water, eating unusual food abroad

Chickweed-Helps control dietary fat metabolism.

Chicory-Reduces stress, anti-inflammatory, protects liver.

Cinnamon-Antioxidant, anti-inflammatory. Studies have shown to be anti-diabetic and aid in heart health.

Cilantro-Rids the body of heavy metals. Lowers anxiety and blood sugar levels.

Comfrey-Pain reliever. Stimulates respiratory system. Helpful with stomach problems, abscesses and wounds.

Corn Silk-Diuretic. Treats urinary tract infections and kidney stones.

Cramp Bark-Uterine sedative and tonic. Good for menses cramps, leg cramps and mild convulsions.

Damiana-Nervous system and sexual stimulant. Strengthens the ovum in women and increases sperm count in men.

Dandelion-Acts as a diuretic without depleting potassium. Kidney and liver support.

Desert Willow-Helps fight infection and aids immune system. Antioxidant and anti-fungal.

Devil's Claw-Arthritis and pain relief. Anti-inflammatory and acts to decrease blood fats, cholesterol and uric acid levels.

Devil's Club-Helps control blood sugar levels. Ginseng-like adaptogen. Treatment of internal and external infections.

Dong Quai-Blood thinner. Used for menopausal symptoms. Sometimes referred to as "female ginseng"

Echinacea-Stimulates white blood cell count. Anti-viral, antibacterial. Good for cold, flu, infections and fevers.

Elderberry-Commonly used for cold and flu relief.

Elecampane-Appetite stimulant. Used for chronic cough and congestion.

Eleuthero-Boosts immunity, reduces fatigue and improves cognition.

Eucalyptus-Antiseptic with antifungal, antiviral, anti-inflammatory and antibacterial properties making it highly effective in treating wounds, minor cuts, acne, boils, insect bites, skin infections.

Eucommia Bark-Strengthens bones and joints. Nervous system tonic.

Eyebright-For bloodshot and irritated eyes. Shrinks swollen sinuses from hay fever.

False Unicorn-Has a reputation for improving fertility in women. Uterine tonic.

Fennel-Aids with gas and stomach cramping.

Feverfew-Used for migraines. Anti-inflammatory.

Fringetree-Liver problems, gallstones, water retention.

Galangal-Has shown cancer fighting properties. Anti-inflammatory. Improves sperm count and function.

Garlic-Lowers cholesterol and triglyceride levels. Anti-microbial. Classic remedy.

Gentian-Taken as a bitter tonic. Stimulates appetite and may help with chronic flatulence.

Ginger-Gas, indigestion, warming sensation and eases nausea.

Ginkgo-Legendary for mental stimulation, concentration, aptitude, memory and alertness. Increases oxygen to the brain.

Ginseng, American-Traditionally used for nervous system stimulation, tones the adrenals, regulates blood pressure and lowers cholesterol. Adaptogen that helps alleviate stress. Known to increase "yin" energy. Has a cooling effect.

Ginseng, Korean-Generally regarded as stronger and opposite to American ginseng. Has warming qualities. Know to increase "yang" energy.

Ginseng, Siberian-Adaptogen. Increases stamina, energy levels, body's resistance to stress, mental alertness and normalizes metabolism.

Goldenseal-Improves digestive issues, antibiotic and immune system booster. Good for urinary tract infections.

Gotu Kola-Cerebral stimulant. Improves circulation. Improves skin.

Grape Seed-Antibacterial, antiviral, anti-inflammatory.

Gravel Root-Diuretic. Aids with kidney stones.

Grindelia-Supports lung and kidney function. Used for asthma relief.

Green Tea-Strong antioxidant. Reduces LDL and can keep blood sugar from rising.

Guarana-Caffeine plant. Nervous system stimulant. Least likely of all caffeine plants to cause anxiety.

Hawthorne- "Cardiotonic herb." Supports healthy heart function. Lowers blood pressure.

Holy Basil-Supports healthy respiratory function. Fights acne. Protects against diabetes. Balances hormones and lowers stress.

Hops-Safe sedative for children and adults. Helpful for nervous stomach and mild pain.

Horehound-Cough relief, digestive aid, motion sickness, bronchitis.

Horny Goat Weed-Helps increase testosterone and estrogen. Natural aphrodisiac.

Horse Chestnut-Strengthens and tones veins. Supports healthy circulatory system.

Horseradish-Stimulant to digestive process. Expels gas and cramping. Used at the early stages of a cold.

Horsetail-Boosts immunity, strengthens bones, powerful antioxidant.

Hyssop-Anti-viral and anti-spasmodic for coughs and asthma. Will induce sweating.

Inmortal-Bronchial dilator and stimulant. Good for lymph drainage in the lungs.

Juniper-Antioxidant. Diuretic.

Kava Kava-Prostate health. Boosts immune system. Strong antioxidant.

Kelp-High vitamin and mineral count. Rich source of iodine.

Kola Nut-Caffeine plant. Minimizes fatigue and promotes alertness. Not to be used long term.

Kudzu-Used for alcohol addiction. Reduces blood pressure, blood sugar and stomach acidity.

Lavender-Used for indigestion, gas, nausea and cramping. Used as an inhalant to ease headaches.

Lemon Balm-Stress reliever. Protects against heart and liver problems. Antibacterial.

Lemon Verbena-Powerful antioxidant. Eases stress.

Licorice-Ulcers, heartburn and infections. Reduces inflammation in stomach lining.

Lily of the Valley-CONSULT A PHYSICIAN. Promotes heart action and increases blood pressure.

Maca Root-Strong antioxidant. Increases energy, mood and memory. Improves female sexual health.

Ma Huang-INTENDED FOR SHORT TERM USE. Treats asthma, cold and flu symptoms. (Also known as Ephedra)

Marshmallow Root-Treats coughs and colds. Digestive system supporter. Repairs gut lining. Fights bacterial infection. Reduces water retention.

Matarique-Decreases the amount of insulin necessary for diabetes. Works on cell membrane permeability to blood sugar.

<u>Milk Thistle</u>-Liver protector and cell regenerator. Prevents free radical damage.

<u>Moringa</u>-Antioxidant, anti-inflammatory. Balances hormones and slows effects of aging. Helps improve digestive health.

Mormon Tea-Similar to Ma Huang but less of a stimulant to the heart, blood pressure and heart rate. Shrinks swollen membranes in the lungs.

Mullein-Respiratory relaxant and bronchial dilator, expands airways and allows freer breathing.   Also used for ear infections.

Myrrh Gum-Used as an anti-bacterial gargle. Topically used to treat swelling.

Nettles-Strong diuretic. Good nutritional supplement...high in iron and calcium.
Noni-Combats inflammation and boosts immunity. Helps reduce cholesterol. Strong antioxidant.

Nux Vomica-Motion sickness, constipation, flu, urinary tract infection.

Oat Seed-Seeds contain anti-inflammatory and tonic to the nervous system.

Ocotillo-Good for glandular and lymphatic swellings and intestinal blockages. Should be used with carrier herbs.

<u>Olive Leaf</u>-Lowers blood pressure, improves cardiovascular health, diabetes, improves brain function.

Oregon Grape Root-Blood purifier. Used for skin condition, constipation and chronic liver malfunction.

Oshá-Bronchial dilator, expectorant and anti-viral agent. Useful in respiratory infections.

Pansy-Popular as a child's alternative to aspirin. Gentle sedative.

Partridge Berry-Useful for difficult periods

Passion Flower-Has been used to treat menopausal symptoms and depression. Lowers blood pressure and reduces anxiety.

Pau D'Arco-Used to treat systemic and yeast infections. Antioxidant. Increases red blood count.

Pennyroyal-Anti-spasmodic. Aids abdominal cramps and helps break up colds.

Pipsissewa-Flushes kidneys and urinary tract. Anti-bacterial.

Poke-Powerful blood purifier and lymph cleanser.

Prickly Ash-Aids with poor circulation. Aids digestion and promotes appetite.

Prickly Poppy-Internally used as a sedative and to reduce pain. Externally used to treat heat rash, hives and other skin irritations.

Propolis-Antifungal, anti-inflammatory and antimicrobial. Used topically for wounds, cold sores and herpes. ***Do not use if you have a bee allergy.***

Psyllium Husk-Used to treat diarrhea and constipation. High in fiber. Helps lower blood sugar and blood pressure.

Pulsatilla-Sedative to promote sleep and ease anxiety.

Red Clover-High mineral content. Mild sedative effects. Helps maintain bone strength. Improves cardiovascular health.

Red Root-Supports immune system and lymphatic strengthener.

Reishi-Regulates blood pressure and eases effects of stress on cardiovascular system. Improves blood flow to the brain, enhances memory and promotes overall vitality and longevity.

Rhodiola-Fights depression and improves brain function. Lowers the hormone cortisol brought on by stress. Supports weight loss.

Saw Palmetto-Hormonal impact on men effecting hair, prostate and kidneys.

Schisandra-Protects liver cells and balances metabolism. Decreases fatigue and boosts immune system. Intensifies mental clarity and alertness. Adjusts stomach acid and lowers blood sugar levels.

Shepherd's Purse-Useful for bladder irritations associated with bleeding and phosphate deposits, used for menstrual hemorrhaging.

Shilajit-Boosts energy, promotes brain health and regulates hormone/immune system.

Skullcap-Calms anxiety and can induce sleep. Reduces inflammation and risk of heart disease. Useful in insomnia, fear, nervous and migraines.

Slippery Elm-Great addition to any IBS diet. Reduces inflammation. Aids in weight loss and lowers stress and anxiety.

Spikenard-Resembles Ginseng in neural-hormonal effect. Strong expectorant.

St. John's Wort-Traditionally used an as antidepressant. Improves mood and regulates hormonal imbalance.

Stillingia-Support the lymphatic system, and it also supports the natural detoxification functions of the mucous membranes, liver and lymphatic tissues. **USE CONSERVATIVELY**

Storksbill-Used to control bleeding. Used mainly in Mexico after childbirth to stem bleeding and to prevent infection.

Thuja-Highly anti-fungal, effective on skin problem (ringworm, jock itch, athlete's foot and candida). Treats urinary tract infection.

Triphala- (Combination of Amia, Haritaki, and Bibhitaki). Highly regarded in Ayurvedic medicine. Cancer fighting properties. Natural colon cleanser. Supports weight loss and low cholesterol. Anti-inflammatory.

Usnea-Similar to penicillin, it can be used for bacterial infections such as strep, staph, TB or yeast but does not affect intestinal flora.

Uva Ursi-Used to treat UTI's, reduce swelling of the bladder, urethra and urinary tract. Also used for bladder and kidney stones.

Valerian-Famously used as a sleep aid. Eases stress and anxiety. Lowers blood pressure.

Vervain-Anti-inflammatory, anti-anxiety and promotes gum health. Antimicrobial and antibacterial.

Virginia Snake Root-Aids constipation, stimulates metabolism and circulation. Increases appetite.

Vitex-AKA Chasteberry. Relieves PMS symptoms, reduces uterine fibroids, improves female fertility.

White Oak-Astringent. Useful for gum inflammation, gingivitis, loose teeth and sore throats. Also used for chronic nosebleeds.

White Willow-Used to relieve headaches, fevers, arthritis and hay fever. Reduces inflammation of joints and tendons.

Wild Cherry Bark-Especially good for dry coughs, asthma and bronchitis.

Wild Sarsaparilla-Called a "Coadaptogen" this will help return an overactive or sluggish system to stasis. Repairs liver and kidney deficiency. Strong antioxidant.

Wild Yam-Regulates blood sugar, eases nausea and improves cholesterol levels.

Witch Hazel-Traditionally used topically for acne, varicose veins and insect bites.

Yarrow-Used for colds, flu, fevers and respiratory infections. Used on wounds to stop bleeding. Mild sedative for anxiety.

Yellow Dock-Blood purifier used for skin problems. Useful for ulcers, constipation and liver congestion.

Yerba Mansa-Very similar to Goldenseal.

Yerba Mate-Tonic, diuretic and stimulant. Said to stimulate muscular and nervous system. Popular as a weight loss aid.

Yerba Santa-Used for colds, laryngitis, bronchitis, hay fever and asthma; famous for all respiratory problems. Will dry up excess fluid in lungs.

Yohimbe-Anxiety, depression erectile dysfunction, exercise performance. USE IN CONSERVATIVE AMOUNTS.

Yucca-Anti-inflammatory for arthritic joints.

HERBAL COMBINATIONS

ALL AID *Greatly stimulates the immune system. Excellent for colds, flu and infections.*

> **Echinacea** Stimulates white blood cell count. Anti-viral, antibacterial.
> **Pau D'Arco** Fortifies the immune system.
> **Usnea** Similar to penicillin without affecting healthy flora in the GI tract.
> **Goldenseal** High anti-bacterial properties.
> **Propolis** Aids damaged tissues from infections.
> **Wild Ginger** Helps break up a cold. Immune system supporter.
> **Cayenne** Facilitates delivery of other herbs. Improves circulation.

ALL AID FOR KIDS Excellent for colds, flu and infections. Slightly syrupy in consistency. Does not contain honey. Best for kids up to 5 or 6 years old.

> **Echinacea** Stimulates white blood cell count. Anti-viral, antibacterial.
> **Burdock** Helps with headaches and keeps the blood from becoming too acidic.
> **Pansy** Child's herbal aspirin.
> **Yarrow** Opens the pores of the skin so toxins can be eliminated.
> **Red Clover** Relieves cough and hyperactivity, which promotes better sleep.
> **Lemon Thyme** Pleasant tasting herb. Greatly enhances the immune system and calms irritability.
> **Marshmallow** Stimulates the immune system to increase white blood cell count.

ALLERGY AID *Use this for hay fever and seasonal allergy symptoms of runny nose and watery eyes. Useful for pollen and animal allergies but no side effects like common antihistamines.*

> **Yerba Santa** Dries up and organizes the mucous membranes of the upper respiratory system.
> **Nettles** Helps the body produce natural antihistamine due to its high chlorophyll count.
> **Eyebright** Reduces eye irritation and nose secretions.
> **Mormon Tea** Shrinks swollen tissue in the nose.

ATHLETES ENDURANCE *This combination increases physical endurance and stamina for peak performance levels, supporting all body systems and increases vitamin absorption.*

Burdock Decreases lactic acid in the joints and muscles. Helps maintain electrolyte balance.
Oshá Helps up oxygen intake and helps eliminate excess carbon dioxide build up in the blood.
Gotu Kola Carries nutrients to the brain, helping to rejuvenate the central nervous system.
Yerba Mansa Inhibits inflammation, infection and tissue injury.
St. John's Wort Mood enhancer. Also, an anti-inflammatory.
American Ginseng Supports the body's ability to handle stresses.
Cayenne Helps carry the other herbs throughout the body and increases the body's ability to move blood to the extremities.

BITTER TONIC *Aids chronic stomach and intestinal problems, gas, heartburn, and burping. Can be taken before a heavy meal, preferably 15 to 30 minutes. Stimulates digestive enzymes.*

Gentian Increases blood supply to the stomach lining and pepsin production.
Cardamom Supports enzyme secretion.
Orange Peel Relieves excess flatulence.

BREATHE DEEPLY *Has therapeutic value in colds, flu, asthma, bronchitis, lung congestion and swollen glands. Useful expectorant.*

Oshá Antiviral to cold and flu. Expectorant and bronchial dilator.
Yerba Mansa Anti-microbial and anti-asthmatic.
Red Root Supports the immune system and helps to clean up metabolic waste.
Pleurisy Traditionally used for chronic infections.
Mullein Respiratory relaxant and bronchial dilator, expands airways and allows freer breathing.

CANDA TONIC *Inhibits candida growth in the intestinal tract, useful in all systemic yeast infections. Also, generally supports the immune system.*

Pau D'Arco Used to treat systemic and yeast infections.
Desert Willow Helps fight infection and aids immune system.
Usnea Inhibits excess yeast infections without effecting healthy flora in the GI tract.
Echinacea Increases white blood cell production and activates the immune response.
Yerba Mansa Prevents the breakdown of the gastrointestinal lining caused by flora imbalance.
Chaparro Amargosa Inhibits candida overgrowth.
Dandelion Relieves excess fluid imbalance in the GI tract created by candida inflammation.

CIRCULATION *Used to strengthen the heart muscle and regulate heart beat as well as helping to remove plaque alone with arterial wall.*

Hawthorne Premier cardiac tonic, strengthens the heart muscle.
Yarrow Strengthens the whole cardiovascular system.
Kelp Provides valuable nutrients and minerals.
Garlic Lowers cholesterol.
Cayenne Promotes healthy circulation.

CLEAR SKIN *Liver and blood cleansing combination. Good for acne, abscesses, psoriasis, scalp irritations, rashes, insect bites and most skin eruptions. Stimulates the liver to increase blood filtration and maintain proper blood pH balance.*

Echinacea Stimulates the immune system's ability to help clean up the blood.
Burdock Resupplies the skin with natural oils.
Yellow Dock Aids fat absorption and decongests the liver.
Oregon Grape Useful for food and skin allergies.
Yarrow Opens the pores of the skin to increase the elimination of waste.
Sarsaparilla Repairs liver deficiency and increases red blood cell count. Mild laxative effects.

CREATIVITY *Increases circulation in the brain thus enhancing memory and the capacity to concentrate.*

> **Ginkgo** Increases mental alertness and aptitude by increasing blood supply and oxygen to the brain.
> **Gotu Kola** Increases neural synapses and carries nutrients through the nervous system, rejuvenating brain cells.
> **Rosemary** Normalizes blood pressure and strengthens capillaries in the head.
> **American Ginseng** Increases nerve fiber growth. General high level adaptogen.
> **Virginia Snake Root** Increases circulation and enhances abilities of other herbs.

ECHINACEA BOMB *Excellent for upper respiratory infections and the first sign of colds, flu and fevers. Soothes sore throat, thins bronchial mucus, antibacterial and anti-viral.*

> **Echinacea** Keeps immune system functioning at its peak, draining the lymphatic system.
> **Oshá** Antiviral to cold and flu. Expectorant and bronchial dilator.
> **Inmortal** Increases secretions to dry sinuses and lungs.
> **Licorice** Dilutes thick mucus making it easier to eliminate.

ENTIRE SYSTEM *This combination stimulates blood circulation toning the whole cardiovascular system and strengthening the liver. It improves cellular function in the brain enhancing memory and mental alertness.*

> **Ginkgo** Increases oxygen to the brain.
> **Hawthorne** Supports healthy heart function. Lowers blood pressure. (Does not work well with beta blockers.)
> **Milk Thistle** Protects liver cells from damage that may be caused by radiation, alcohol and chemicals.
> **American Ginseng** Lowers high blood sugar and elevated uric acid. Helps the body fight long term stress.
> **Virginia Snake Root** Increases absorption of vitamins A, D and E and dietary fats.
> **Gotu Kola** Aids sluggish metabolism and increases blood flow to the brain.
> **Nettles** High in chlorophyll, high in nutritional content.
> **Cayenne** Acts to carry the other herbs through the body.

ESSENTIAL SUPPLEMENTS *Replaces minerals depleted in the body depleted by everyday stress. Contains iron, calcium, iodine, potassium, phosphorus and silica. Reduces loss of electrolytes.*

Alfalfa Nutritive herb that has a high mineral content that is easily digestible, particularly calcium, vitamin K, and folic acid.
Kelp Sea vegetable with high calcium content.
Yellow Dock Releases stored iron in the liver and increases assimilation of dietary fats.
Nettles High in chlorophyll, iron and calcium. Premier blood builder.
Wild Sarsaparilla Called a "Coadaptogen" this will help return an overactive or sluggish system to stasis. Repairs liver and kidney deficiency. Strong antioxidant.

GET YOU GOING *Reviving formula that increases circulation and boosts the adrenals. Contains caffeine.*

Guarana Nervous system stimulant. Least likely of all caffeine plants to cause anxiety.
Kola Nut Supplies blood to the skeletal muscles and is mildly hypertensive.
Damiana Nervous system stimulant.
Virginia Snake Root Blood and nervous system stimulant.

GINSENG FLING *Premier constitutional tonic with apoptogenic properties giving the body improved ability to adapt to stresses of life.*

American Ginseng Traditionally used for nervous system stimulation, tones the adrenals, regulates blood pressure and lowers cholesterol. Adaptogen that helps alleviate stress.
Ginseng, Siberian-Adaptogen. Increases stamina, energy levels, body's resistance to stress, mental alertness and normalizes metabolism.
Licorice Supports exhausted adrenals.
Motherwort Relaxes the blood vessels.
Oat Seed Aids nervous exhaustion.
Devil's Claw Anti-inflammatory and lowers amount of hormones needed by the body daily.

GUM HEALTH *Promoting healthy gums and mouth, good for gingivitis, sore throats, swollen lymph nodes and strep throat. Can be used as a gargle and swallowed.*

Propolis Antifungal, anti-inflammatory and antimicrobial.
Myrrh Gum Stimulates immune response to infections.
Spearmint Taste…trust me.

IMMUNE SUPPORT *Deeply replenishes the immune system and acts as preventative.*

Astragalus Strong anti-inflammatory, immune booster, antioxidant.
Reishi Has been shown to assist the immune system in preventing tumors and attacking malignant cells.
Cat's Claw Decreases fatigue. Relieves depression and enhances immune function.
Red Root Supports the immune system and helps to clean up metabolic waste.
Burdock Alkalinizes and eliminates toxins in the bloodstream.
Siberian Ginseng Supports longevity and endurance levels.

LIMB SUPPORT *May increase joint mobility and expand range of motion for sore, stiff joints and muscles. Decreases urea and lactic acid due to inflammation resulting in lowering inflammation.*

Devil's Claw Arthritis and pain relief. Anti-inflammatory and acts to decrease blood fats, cholesterol and uric acid levels.
Yucca Relieves pain in the joints.
Yerba Mansa Inhibits inflammation, infection and tissue injury.
Burdock Keeps the blood clean.
Alfalfa Alkalinizes an acidic blood stream and replaces lost nutrients.
Cayenne Increases blood support.

LYMPH LUBE *Used for tonsillitis, swollen glands, enlarged spleen, lymphatic congestion, infections and inflammations. Stimulates immune response by supporting the lymphatic system.*

Red Root Supports immune system and lymphatic strengthener.
Burdock Alkalizes pH and supports liver to cleanse the body relieving waste products from inflammations.
Echinacea Antibacterial, stimulates white blood cells to an area of infection and speeds up a slow healing process.
Yerba Mansa Decreases inflammation and reduces tissue damage in injured cells.
Ocotillo Specifically drains the lymph in the pelvis proving value for intestinal infections.
Stillingia Supports the lymphatic system, and it also supports the natural detoxification functions of the mucous membranes, liver and lymphatic tissues.
USE CONSERVATIVELY
Blue Flag Powerful liver lymphatic, increases the body's metabolism.

LIVER SUPPORT *For poor digestion aggravated by fats, alcohol or coffee, it helps with hangovers. Helps as a detox.*

Echinacea Stimulates blood cleansing abilities of the immune system and controls septic conditions that liver congestion can cause.
Barberry Increases the liver's ability to breakdown hydrocarbons and other toxins that otherwise get stored in the liver.
Toadflax Specific for tiredness that's associated with liver backlog of catabolic wastes.
Fringetree Relieves mild liver pain associated with bile blockage and nausea.
Dandelion Blood alkalinizer and helps blood circulate through the liver.
Blue Flag Aids those with the inability to digest food well.

MALE VITALITY *Increases male virility by supporting the reproductive organs and strengthening prostate function and testosterone levels.*

Dong Quai Increases steroidal binding sites to testosterone sensitive cells, for prostate and testicular deficiencies, helping balance the hormones.
Saw Palmetto Helps nourish the tissues of the male reproductive system, specifically the prostate.
American Ginseng Helps reduce hormonal imbalances.
Wild Sarsaparilla Specific for benign prostatic hypertrophy with poor steroid production.
Virginia Snake Root Helps the body absorb dietary oil and vitamins, aids circulation.

MELLOW MELLOW *Relaxes, calms and tones the nerves. Has antispasmodic properties to muscles and organs. Good for insomnia, anxiety and muscle twitching.*

Skullcap Calms anxiety and can induce sleep.
Passion Flower Muscle relaxant and mild sedative.
Hops Helpful for nervous stomach and mild pain.
St. John's Wort For stress induced agitation and depression.
American Ginseng Helps with stress.

MENSTRUAL AID *Used for chronic menses pain, discharge, excessive bleeding or irregular periods. Supports reproductive organs and helps regulate periods to be on time.*

Aletris Relieves constipation and gas.
Partridge Berry Supports the whole reproductive system and quiets nervous irritability and reduces bloating.
Blue Cohosh Specific for the heavy sensation and cramping. Also aids a slow starting cycle.
Cramp Bark Alleviates pain that runs through the sacral and leg area. Muscle relaxant.

METAL CLEANSE *Acts to leach heavy metals and toxicity from the thyroid, blood and liver. Protects the liver from further damage.*

> **Milk Thistle** Liver protector and cell regenerator. Prevents free radical damage.
> **Burdock** Blood cleanser. Reduces uric acid.
> **Kelp** Electrolyte supporter. Decongests the thyroid.
> **Blue Flag** Supports an overworked liver. Stimulates immune function.

NAUSEA CALM *Good for morning sickness, motion sickness and general nausea. Recommended to mix in drink or juice.*

> **Wild Yam** Calms cramps and sudden nausea.
> **Cramp Bark** Relaxes the diaphragm and stomach contractions.
> **Wild Ginger** Antispasmodic that warms the stomach.
> **Peppermint** Aids digestion and sweetens formula.

PICK ME UP *Produces a feeling of well being for those experiencing "the blues." Oxygenizes the brain to think clearer and nourishes the nervous system.*

> **Kava Kava** Aids in relaxing the body yet increases communicativeness.
> **St John's Wort** Helps with agitation, depression, nervous exhaustion and anxiety.
> **Passion Flower** Mood elevator, enhances circulation.
> **Ginkgo** Useful in impaired cerebral blood supply.
> **Kelp** Excellent mineral replacer for nervous system nutrients.
> **Lavender** Known for its calming properties.
> **Oat Seed** Deep neural tonic and restorative.
> **American Ginseng** Premier adaptogen, supports stress induced nervous system disorders.

PRE-MENSTRUAL AID *This combination is good for PMS and irregular periods. Helps balance estrogen/progesterone levels.*

> **Vitex** Relieves PMS symptoms, may reduce uterine fibroids.
> **Black Haw** Reduces clotting and relieves painful periods and low back pain.
> **Raspberry** Supports the function of Vitex.
> **Dandelion** Reduces bloating and water retention.

REJUVENATE *Promotes longevity, induces mental clarity and cleanses the system.*

    Astragalus Strengthens the body's resistance to illness. Strong immune system tonic.
Gotu Kola Improves thyroid function and slow metabolism.
Virginia Snake Root Increases poor dietary vitamin absorption. Induces sweating.
Nettles Alkalinizing diuretic. Mineral replacer. High in chlorophyll and useful with allergies.
American Ginseng Adaptogen. Supports the overall adrenal function.
Cayenne Facilitates blood movement.

SLEEP AID *For restless and nervousness. Aids insomnia. Helps to fall asleep faster and sleep deeper.*

    Valerian Used to fall asleep quicker and stay asleep longer.
Hops Alleviates muscle spasms and cramps.
Skullcap Calms anxiety and induces sleep.

URINARY AID I *Aids in relieving active infections of the urinary tract, it will soothe and cool out the kidney, bladder and urethra.*

    Marshmallow Immune stimulant. Soothes inflammations and absorbs toxins.
Aspen Similar to aspirin. Reduces fever, pain and inflammation.
Yerba Mansa Lowers acid levels. Helps reduce damage to swollen tissue.
Pipsissewa Flushes kidneys and urinary tract.
Corn Silk Traditionally used in chronic bladder infections. Increases urine output.
Horsetail Relieves irritation and aids with acute inflammation.

URINARY AID II *For low grade urinary infections. Also stimulates and acts as preventative.*

    Pipsissewa Flushes kidneys and urinary tract.
Myrrh Gum Increases red blood cell count and activates immune system.
Juniper Antioxidant. Diuretic.
Agrimony Useful in urinary tract infections.
Corn Silk Traditionally used in chronic bladder infections. Increases urine output.

ORGAN SYSTEM DISORDERS

This section aims to give you a generalized synopsis of health problems and the traditional herbal remedies for them. It is categorized by the organ system and meant to be general. Diet, exercise and other factors play into individual pathologies. Herbs can act as a facilitator in the healing process but do not consider these pages a diagnosis. As always, please consult a physician, clinical herbalist or naturopath.

RESPIRATORY-sinuses, throat & lungs

Asthma
  Humid-Elecampane, Horehound, Yerba Mansa, Yerba Santa, Grindelia, Breathe Deep
  Dry-Inmortal, Pleurisy

Bronchitis
  Acute-Breathe Deeply, Echinacea, Slippery Elm
  Chronic-Elecampane, Spikenard, Prickly Ash, Horehound, Grindelia
  Dry-Inmortal, Pleurisy

Coughs-Slippery Elm, Red Clover, Grindelia, Wild Cherry, Horehound
  Dry-Oshá, Lobelia, Pleurisy

Hay Fever-Allergy Aid, Echinacea, Nettles, All Aid

Head Cold-Inmortal, Yerba Mansa, Ginger, All Aid

Flu-Spikenard, Oshá, All Aid, Echinacea, Yerba Mansa, Propolis, Black Cohosh

Laryngitis-Slippery Elm, Marshmallow

Sinusitis-Inmortal, Yerba Mansa, Goldenseal, Ma Huang (caution), Mormon Tea, Eyebright, Baptisia, Grindelia

Sore/Strep Throat-Gum Toner, Red Root, Echinacea, Slippery Elm,

Tonsillitis-Red Root, Oshá, Goldenseal, Yerba Mansa, Echinacea, Myrrh Gum, Baptisia

<u>GASTROINTESTINAL-mouth, esophagus, stomach, small and large intestines</u>

Canker Sores (Mouth)-Echinacea, Dandelion, Burdock, Gum Toner, Myrrh Gum (gargle)

Colic-Peppermint, Wild Yam

Colitis-Peppermint Oil, Marshmallow, Echinacea

Constipation-Cascara Sagrada, Bitter Tonic

Diarrhea-White Oak Bark

Gastritis-Marshmallow, Calendula, Yerba Mansa

Hemorrhoids-Cascara Sagrada, Bitter Tonic

Herpes-Yerba Mansa, Motherwort, Burdock
>   **Topical**-Goldenseal, Yerba Mansa, White Oak Bark, Propolis

Hiccups-Peppermint, Black Haw

Indigestion-Gentian, Bitter Tonic

Heartburn-Blue Vervain

Gas-Cinnamon, Bitter Tonic

Nausea-Ginger, Wild Yam, Nausea Calm

Parasites-Black Walnut, Garlic, Chaparro Amargosa

Stomach Flu-Oshá, Echinacea, Marshmallow

Ulcers-Marshmallow, Licorice

Vomiting-Chamomile, Mint, Wild Yam

<u>LIVER AND GALLBLADDER</u>

General Support-Fringetree, Celandine, Yarrow, Wild Yam

Cirrhosis-Milk Thistle, Celandine, Licorice

Hepatitis-Milk Thistle, Fringetree, Licorice

Jaundice-Milk Thistle, Oregon Grape Root, Barberry, Fringetree, Dandelion

<u>HEART AND BLOOD VESSELS</u>

Hypertension-Hawthorne, Yarrow, Passion Flower, Garlic, *Circulation*

Hypotension-Hawthorne, *Circulation*, Licorice

Palpitations-Hawthorne, Motherwort, *Circulation*

Varicose Veins-Ginkgo, St. John's Wort, Horse Chestnut
　　　Topical-Witch Hazel

<u>ENDOCRINE/METABOLIC-adrenals, thyroid, pancreas</u>

Adrenal Exhaustion-American Ginseng, Siberian Ginseng, Licorice

Hypoglycemia-American Ginseng, Devil's Club, Cayenne, Prickly Ash

Diabetes/Hyperglycemia-Brickellia, American Ginseng, Matarique, Blueberry, Burdock

Hypothyroid-Gotu Kola, Oregon Grape, Passion Flower, Virginia Snake Root

Hyperthyroid-Motherwort

Obesity-Nettles, Guarana, Kola Nut, Chickweed

<u>IMMUNE/LYMPHATIC</u>

Fevers-Echinacea, Elder, Yarrow

Infections-Echinacea, Myrrh Gum, *Lymph Lube, All Aid*
　　　Fungal-Usnea, *Canda Tonic*, Pau D'Arco, Desert Willow

Mono-Echinacea, Usnea, Red Root, Ocotillo, *Lymph Lube, Immune Support*

Support-Astragalus, Reishi, Burdock, Virginia Snake Root, Baptisia, *Lymph Lube, Immune Support, Rejuvenate*

<h1 style="text-align:center"><u>REPRODUCTIVE</u></h1>

Candida-Pau D'Arco, Desert Willow, Usnea, Chaparral, Echinacea, *Canda-Tonic*

Cervicitis-Raspberry, Partridge Berry, Dong Quai, False Unicorn, Calendula (douche), Echinacea (suppository)

Cramps-Blue Cohosh, Dong Quai, Wild Yam, Cramp Bark, Black Haw

Cysts-Red Root, Chaparral, Dong Quai

Endometriosis-Vitex, Black Cohosh, *Pre-Menstrual Aid*

Fibroids-Red Root, Ocotillo, Vitex

Irregular Periods-*Menstrual Aid,* Raspberry, Dong Quai (during estrogen phase), Vitex (during progesterone phase)

Menopause-Dong Quai, False Unicorn

PMS-Vitex, Motherwort, Passion flower, *Pre-Menstrual Aid*

Prostatitis-Saw Palmetto, Yerba Mansa, Dong Quai, *Male Vitality*

Vaginitis-Echinacea, Yerba Mansa, Black Cohosh

<h1 style="text-align:center"><u>SKIN, HAIR, EYES AND EARS</u></h1>

Abscess (Infection)-Echinacea, Cleaver, Yellow Dock
 Topical-Calendula, Comfrey, Thuja
 Fungal-Usnea, Myrrh Gum

Acne-Oregon Grape Root, Yellow Dock, Dandelion, Burdock, *Clear Skin*

Eczema-Burdock, Cleavers, Oregon Grape root, Devil's Club, Pleurisy, *Clear Skin*
 Topical-Grindelia

Herpes-Goldenseal, Yerba Mansa, Calendula, Oat seed, St. John's Wort, Dong Quai
 Topical-Echinacea, Myrrh Gum

Insect Bites-**Topical**-Echinacea

Poison Ivy/Oak-Grindelia, White Oak Bark

Psoriasis-Burdock, Yellow Dock, Cleavers, Oat seed, *Clear Skin*

Tinnitus-Pulsatilla, Ginkgo

Tired Eyes-Blueberry, Eyebright

NERVOUS SYSTEM AND PAIN

Anxiety-Motherwort, Pulsatilla, *Mellow Mellow*

Depression-St. John's Wort, Passion Flower, *Pick Me Up*

Insomnia-Passion Flower, Skullcap, Hops, Valerian, *Sleep Aid*

Mental Alertness-Ginkgo, Gotu Kola, *Creativity*

Pain-
    General-Black Cohosh, Prickly Poppy, Valerian, Aspen

Hangover-Oregon grape root, Guarana, Chaparral, Toadlax
    Sciatica-Skullcap

Headaches-Skullcap, Feverfew, Valerian, Guarana, Passion Flower

URINARY TRACT

Cystitis/Urethritis-Yerba Mansa, Agrimony, Pipsissewa, *Urinary Aid I & II*

Incontinence-Corn Silk, Horsetail, Agrimony

Pain-Marshmallow, Kava, White Willow, Aspen

Stones-Shepherd's Purse, Gravel root

MUSCULO-SKELETAL (includes connective tissue)

Arthritis-Devi's Claw, Yucca, *Limb Support*, Nettles

Bruises/Sprains, Breaks-Black Cohosh, Comfrey
    Topical-Arnica, St. John's Wort

Gout-Shepherd's Purse, Devi's Claw

Rheumatism-Black Cohosh, Echinacea, Devil's Claw, Feverfew, *Limb Support*
    Topical-Wintergreen

Tendonitis/Bursitis-Echinacea, Prickly Ash

CHILDREN

Colic-Anise, Chamomile

Diaper Rash-Marshmallow

Diarrhea-Peppermint

Ear Infections-Echinacea

Fever-Echinacea, Elder, Yarrow, Pansy

Headache-Burdock, Skullcap

Teething-Chamomile, Passion Flower

Vomiting-Lavender, Peppermint, Slippery Elm

Notes on Alternate Preparations

Tinctures are a preferred form for bitter medicinals; the taste can be disguised in juice or sweetened. Tinctures provide a quick assimilation and easy dosage monitoring. Many herbs contain compounds that aren't easily given up in water-based deliveries such as tea and many bulk herbs can lose potency. Tincturing fresh herbs is a great way to ensure a long shelf life by using alcohol as a preserver. The term "extract" can mean any strength however a standardized **ratio of 1:5 herb to liquid with anywhere from 40 to 95% alcohol** is widely used. 15-20 drops of extract are equivalent to a #0 capsule, 25-30 drops are equivalent to a #00 capsule. There are numerous websites and communities dedicated to the extraction and bottling of tinctures. I recommend doing more research before attempting.

Teas have advantages and have been used for centuries. Hot teas can also facilitate sweating when coupled with diaphoretic herbs. Larger amounts of vitamins, minerals and enzymes can be extracted with longer steeping of nutritional water-soluble herbs.

Capsules, when purchased from reputable vendors, they often contain high quality plant material. To prepare capsules, simply grind the dried roots, leaves or blooms of the plant and fill capsules with the resulting powder. You can grind dried plants with an old-fashioned mortar and pestle or try using an electric blender or coffee mill. Capsules are inexpensive and available in many health food stores; one 00-sized capsule can hold about 500 milligrams of a dried herb but weigh your own to get an exact measurement.